DR. BARBARA O'NEILL CURE FOR ARTHRITIS

Achieve Optimal Wellness, Cure Arthritis Naturally Through Dr. Barbara Approved Remedies, Diets And Non-Toxic Lifestyle

Dr. Frank Douglas

Table of Contents

CHAPTER 1

Dr. Barbara O'Neill Cure for Arthritis: Introduction to Dr. Barbara O'Neill and Arthritis

Arthritis is a common and often debilitating condition affecting millions of people worldwide. Understanding the causes, symptoms, and treatments for arthritis is crucial for managing this disease effectively. Dr. Barbara O'Neill, a renowned health practitioner and naturopath, has developed a comprehensive approach to managing arthritis through natural remedies and dietary adjustments. This guide delves into her philosophy, the nature of arthritis, and the power of natural and herbal treatments in alleviating arthritis symptoms.

Dr. Barbara O'Neill's Journey and Philosophy

Dr. Barbara O'Neill's journey into natural health and healing began with her personal experiences and academic pursuits. With a background in biochemistry and naturopathy, Dr. O'Neill combines scientific knowledge with natural health principles. She has dedicated her career to educating people about the benefits of natural remedies, emphasizing the body's ability to heal itself when given the right tools.

Dr. O'Neill's philosophy revolves around holistic health, focusing on the interconnectedness of the body, mind, and spirit. She believes that a balanced diet, proper hydration, regular physical activity, and natural remedies can significantly improve overall health and manage chronic conditions like arthritis. Her approach is patient-centric, empowering individuals to take control of their health through informed choices and natural therapies.

Understanding Arthritis: Types, Symptoms, and Causes

Arthritis is a term that encompasses over 100 different types of joint diseases and conditions. The most common forms are osteoarthritis (OA) and rheumatoid arthritis (RA).

- **Osteoarthritis (OA):** This is a degenerative joint disease primarily affecting older adults. It occurs when the cartilage that cushions the ends of bones in the joints wears down over time, leading to pain, stiffness, and decreased mobility.

- **Rheumatoid Arthritis (RA):** RA is an autoimmune disorder where the immune system mistakenly attacks the synovium (the lining of the membranes that surround the joints), causing inflammation, pain, and swelling. Over time, RA can result in joint deformity and bone erosion.

Common Symptoms of Arthritis:

- Joint pain and stiffness

- Swelling and tenderness in the affected areas

- Reduced range of motion

- Redness around the joints

- Fatigue, particularly in RA

- Fever (in autoimmune forms like RA)

Causes of Arthritis:

- **Genetic Factors:** Family history can increase the risk of certain types of arthritis.

- **Age:** The risk of developing most types of arthritis increases with age.

- **Sex:** Women are more likely to develop RA, while men are more prone to gout.

- **Injuries:** Joint injuries can cause or exacerbate arthritis.

- **Obesity:** Excess weight puts additional stress on joints, particularly the knees, hips, and spine.

- **Infections:** Some bacterial and viral infections can trigger arthritis.

Diet plays a critical role in managing arthritis. Certain foods can exacerbate inflammation, while others can help reduce it. Dr. Barbara O'Neill emphasizes the importance of an anti-inflammatory diet rich in fruits, vegetables, whole grains, lean proteins, and healthy fats.

Anti-Inflammatory Foods:

- **Fruits and Vegetables:** Rich in antioxidants, these foods help combat inflammation. Berries, leafy greens, and cruciferous vegetables like broccoli are particularly beneficial.

- **Omega-3 Fatty Acids:** Found in fish like salmon and flaxseeds, omega-3s reduce inflammation and joint pain.

- **Whole Grains:** Foods like oats, quinoa, and brown rice provide fiber and nutrients that support overall health.

- **Nuts and Seeds:** These are good sources of healthy fats and protein.

- **Herbs and Spices:** Turmeric, ginger, and garlic have potent anti-inflammatory properties.

Foods to Avoid:

- **Processed Foods:** High in trans fats and sugars, these can increase inflammation.

- **Red Meat:** Often contains saturated fats that can exacerbate inflammation.

- **Refined Carbohydrates:** Foods like white bread and pastries can spike blood sugar levels and increase inflammation.

The Power of Herbs in Treating Arthritis

Introduction to Herbal Medicine

Herbal medicine, or phytotherapy, uses plant-based substances for therapeutic purposes. Herbs have been used for centuries to treat various ailments, including arthritis. Dr. Barbara O'Neill advocates for incorporating specific herbs into daily routines to help manage arthritis symptoms naturally and effectively.

Benefits of Using Natural Remedies for Arthritis

1. Reduced Side Effects: Unlike many pharmaceutical treatments, natural remedies typically have fewer side effects. **2. Holistic Approach:** Natural remedies often address the root cause of symptoms rather than just masking them. **3. Cost-Effective:** Many natural treatments are less expensive than prescription medications.

Safety and Efficacy of Herbal Treatments

While natural remedies can be highly effective, it's crucial to use them correctly. Dosage and preparation methods can significantly impact their efficacy. Consulting with a healthcare provider or a qualified naturopath like Dr. O'Neill is essential to ensure safety and proper use.

Herbal Remedies for Arthritis

1. Turmeric (Curcuma longa): Turmeric contains curcumin, a compound with potent anti-inflammatory and antioxidant properties. It can help reduce pain and improve joint function.

Dosage and How to Use:

- **Supplement Form:** Take 500-1,000 mg of curcumin per day, divided into two doses.

- **Turmeric Tea:** Boil 1 teaspoon of turmeric powder in 2 cups of water. Simmer for 10 minutes, strain, and add honey or lemon to taste. Drink twice daily.

2. Ginger (Zingiber officinale): Ginger has anti-inflammatory properties that can help reduce arthritis symptoms. It can be consumed fresh, dried, or in supplement form.

Dosage and How to Use:

- **Fresh Ginger:** Chew a small piece of fresh ginger daily or add it to smoothies and salads.

- **Ginger Tea:** Slice a 1-inch piece of ginger root and steep it in hot water for 10 minutes. Drink 2-3 cups daily.

- **Supplement Form:** Take 250 mg of ginger extract 2-3 times daily.

3. Boswellia (Boswellia serrata): Also known as Indian frankincense, Boswellia has been shown to reduce inflammation and pain in arthritis.

Dosage and How to Use:

- **Supplement Form:** Take 300-500 mg of Boswellia extract 2-3 times daily.

- **Boswellia Tea:** Steep 1 teaspoon of Boswellia resin in hot water for 10 minutes. Drink twice daily.

4. Devil's Claw (Harpagophytum procumbens): Devil's Claw is effective in reducing pain and inflammation in arthritis.

Dosage and How to Use:

- **Supplement Form:** Take 600-1,200 mg of Devil's Claw extract per day, divided into two doses.

- **Devil's Claw Tea:** Boil 1 teaspoon of dried Devil's Claw root in 2 cups of water for 15 minutes. Strain and drink twice daily.

5. Willow Bark (Salix alba): Willow bark contains salicin, which is similar to aspirin and has pain-relieving and anti-inflammatory effects.

Dosage and How to Use:

- **Supplement Form:** Take 120-240 mg of willow bark extract daily.

- **Willow Bark Tea:** Steep 1 teaspoon of dried willow bark in hot water for 10 minutes. Drink 2-3 times daily.

6. Eucalyptus (Eucalyptus globulus): Eucalyptus oil can be used topically to reduce pain and inflammation in arthritis.

Dosage and How to Use:

- **Eucalyptus Oil Massage:** Mix a few drops of eucalyptus oil with a carrier oil (like coconut or olive oil) and massage into the affected joints twice daily.

- **Eucalyptus Bath:** Add a few drops of eucalyptus oil to a warm bath and soak for 15-20 minutes.

7. Cat's Claw (Uncaria tomentosa): Cat's Claw has anti-inflammatory properties and can help improve immune function.

Dosage and How to Use:

- **Supplement Form:** Take 250-350 mg of Cat's Claw extract daily.

- **Cat's Claw Tea:** Boil 1 teaspoon of dried Cat's Claw root in 2 cups of water for 10 minutes. Strain and drink twice daily.

Incorporating Natural Remedies into Your Routine

To effectively manage arthritis with natural remedies, consistency is key. Here are some tips for incorporating these remedies into your daily routine:

- **Create a Schedule:** Set specific times for taking supplements or preparing teas to ensure you don't miss doses.

- **Combine Remedies:** Use a combination of dietary changes, herbal supplements, and topical treatments for a comprehensive approach.

- **Monitor Progress:** Keep a journal of your symptoms and any changes you notice. This can help you identify which remedies are most effective for you.

- **Stay Hydrated:** Drinking plenty of water is essential for overall health and can help improve the efficacy of natural treatments.

CHAPTER 2

Dr. Barbara O'Neill Cure for Arthritis: Turmeric and Ginger Anti-Inflammatory Blend

Arthritis is a debilitating condition that affects millions of people worldwide. Characterized by inflammation of the joints, it can cause severe pain, stiffness, and reduced mobility. While there are various treatments available, many people are turning to natural remedies for relief. Dr. Barbara O'Neill, a renowned naturopath and health educator, has extensively researched and recommended natural treatments for arthritis, emphasizing the anti-inflammatory properties of certain herbs and spices. Two of the most potent ingredients in this regard are turmeric and ginger.

Recipe: Golden Milk with Turmeric and Ginger

Golden Milk, also known as Turmeric Milk, is a traditional Ayurvedic drink that has been used for centuries to promote health and well-being. It is particularly beneficial for its anti-inflammatory properties, which can help in reducing arthritis symptoms. Here's how to prepare it:

Ingredients:

- 1 cup of milk (dairy or plant-based such as almond, coconut, or oat milk)
- 1 teaspoon of turmeric powder
- 1/2 teaspoon of ginger powder (or 1-inch piece of fresh ginger, grated)
- 1/4 teaspoon of cinnamon powder
- 1 tablespoon of honey or maple syrup (optional, for sweetness)
- A pinch of black pepper (to enhance the absorption of curcumin, the active ingredient in turmeric)
- A pinch of cardamom or nutmeg (optional, for additional flavor)

Instructions:

1. **Heat the Milk:** Pour the milk into a small saucepan and place it over medium heat.
2. **Add the Spices:** Add the turmeric, ginger, cinnamon, black pepper, and optional cardamom or nutmeg to the milk.
3. **Simmer:** Stir the mixture continuously and bring it to a gentle simmer. Do not let it boil. Simmer for about 5-10 minutes until the spices are well blended.
4. **Sweeten (Optional):** Remove the saucepan from the heat and add honey or maple syrup if desired.
5. **Strain and Serve:** If using fresh ginger, strain the milk to remove the pieces. Pour into a cup and serve warm.

Dosage and How to Use:

- **Dosage:** Drink one cup of Golden Milk once or twice a day. It is best consumed in the morning to start your day with a boost of anti-inflammatory compounds or in the evening as a soothing drink before bedtime.
- **Usage Duration:** Consistent use over several weeks can provide noticeable relief from arthritis symptoms. However, always consult with a healthcare provider before starting any new treatment regimen.

How Turmeric and Ginger Help in Reducing Arthritis Inflammation

Turmeric: Turmeric contains a powerful compound called curcumin, which has been extensively studied for its anti-inflammatory and antioxidant properties. Curcumin works by inhibiting several molecules that play a role in inflammation, including nuclear factor kappa-light-chain-enhancer of activated B cells (NF-kB) and cyclooxygenase-2 (COX-2). These molecules are known to be involved in the inflammatory process seen in arthritis.

Benefits of Turmeric in Arthritis:

- **Reduces Joint Inflammation:** Curcumin has been shown to reduce inflammation in the joints, alleviating pain and improving joint function.
- **Antioxidant Effects:** Turmeric's antioxidant properties help neutralize free radicals, which can cause oxidative stress and damage to joint tissues.
- **Modulates Immune Response:** Curcumin can help modulate the immune system, reducing autoimmune responses that contribute to conditions like rheumatoid arthritis.

Ginger: Ginger is another powerful anti-inflammatory agent that can be highly beneficial for arthritis sufferers. It contains bioactive compounds such as gingerol, which have been shown to reduce inflammation and pain.

Benefits of Ginger in Arthritis:

- **Reduces Pain and Stiffness:** Studies have found that ginger can significantly reduce pain and stiffness in people with osteoarthritis and rheumatoid arthritis.
- **Inhibits Inflammatory Pathways:** Ginger inhibits several inflammatory pathways, including the production of prostaglandins and leukotrienes, which are involved in the inflammatory response.
- **Enhances Circulation:** Ginger improves blood circulation, which can help reduce swelling and inflammation in the joints.

Combined Effects of Turmeric and Ginger: When used together, turmeric and ginger offer a synergistic effect, enhancing each other's anti-inflammatory properties. This combination can provide more substantial relief from arthritis symptoms than either herb alone.

Scientific Evidence: Several clinical studies support the use of turmeric and ginger for arthritis. For instance, a study published in the Journal of Medicinal Food found that patients with osteoarthritis who took a ginger extract experienced significant reductions in knee pain and other symptoms. Similarly, research published in the Journal of Clinical

Rheumatology demonstrated that curcumin was as effective as nonsteroidal anti-inflammatory drugs (NSAIDs) in reducing arthritis symptoms without the associated side effects.

Boswellia Serrata Tea

Boswellia Serrata, also known as Indian Frankincense, is another potent natural remedy for arthritis. It has been used in traditional Ayurvedic medicine for centuries due to its powerful anti-inflammatory properties. Boswellia Serrata contains boswellic acids, which inhibit the production of pro-inflammatory enzymes, thereby reducing inflammation and pain.

Recipe: Boswellia Serrata Herbal Tea

Boswellia Serrata can be consumed as an herbal tea to help manage arthritis symptoms. Here's how to prepare it:

Ingredients:

- 1 teaspoon of Boswellia Serrata powder
- 1 cup of hot water
- Honey or lemon (optional, for taste)

Instructions:

1. **Heat Water:** Boil one cup of water.
2. **Add Boswellia Serrata Powder:** Add the Boswellia Serrata powder to the hot water.
3. **Steep:** Allow the mixture to steep for 10-15 minutes.
4. **Strain and Serve:** Strain the tea to remove any sediment and pour it into a cup. Add honey or lemon if desired.

Dosage and How to Use:

- **Dosage:** Drink one cup of Boswellia Serrata tea once or twice a day.
- **Usage Duration:** Regular consumption over several weeks is recommended to see noticeable improvements in arthritis symptoms. Consultation with a healthcare provider is advised before starting this regimen.

Benefits of Boswellia Serrata in Managing Arthritis Pain

Anti-Inflammatory Properties: Boswellia Serrata's primary benefit in arthritis management comes from its anti-inflammatory properties. The boswellic acids in Boswellia inhibit the enzyme 5-lipoxygenase (5-LO), which is involved in the production of leukotrienes. Leukotrienes are molecules that cause inflammation, particularly in autoimmune diseases like rheumatoid arthritis.

Benefits of Boswellia Serrata in Arthritis:

- **Reduces Joint Pain:** Boswellia has been shown to significantly reduce joint pain and improve mobility in people with arthritis.
- **Decreases Swelling:** The anti-inflammatory effects help decrease swelling in the joints.
- **Prevents Cartilage Loss:** Some studies suggest that Boswellia can help prevent the breakdown of cartilage, which is a major issue in osteoarthritis.
- **Improves Physical Function:** Regular use of Boswellia Serrata can lead to improved physical function and quality of life for arthritis sufferers.

Scientific Evidence: Research supports the efficacy of Boswellia Serrata in managing arthritis. For example, a study published in Phytomedicine found that patients with osteoarthritis of the knee experienced significant reductions in pain and improvements in knee flexion and walking distance after taking a Boswellia extract. Another study in the International Journal of Phytotherapy and Phytopharmacology reported similar benefits in patients with rheumatoid arthritis, highlighting Boswellia's potential to reduce pain and inflammation without the side effects commonly associated with NSAIDs.

Synergistic Use with Other Anti-Inflammatory Herbs: Boswellia Serrata can be used in combination with other anti-inflammatory herbs such as turmeric and ginger for enhanced effects. This multi-faceted approach can provide comprehensive relief from arthritis symptoms, leveraging the unique properties of each herb.

Practical Tips for Use:

- **Consistency is Key:** Regular and consistent use is essential to experience the full benefits. Incorporate Boswellia Serrata tea into your daily routine for optimal results.
- **Complementary Therapies:** Consider using Boswellia Serrata alongside other natural treatments such as turmeric and ginger, as well as lifestyle modifications like a balanced diet and regular exercise.
- **Monitoring and Adjustment:** Pay attention to how your body responds to the tea and adjust the dosage if necessary. Always consult with a healthcare professional before making any significant changes to your treatment plan.

In conclusion, the use of natural remedies like turmeric, ginger, and Boswellia Serrata offers a promising approach to managing arthritis symptoms. These herbs provide potent anti-inflammatory effects that can help reduce pain, swelling, and improve joint function. By incorporating these remedies into your daily routine, you can take proactive steps towards better managing arthritis and improving your overall quality of life.

CHAPTER 3

Recipe: Willow Bark Decoction

Willow bark, often referred to as "nature's aspirin," has been used for centuries as a natural remedy for pain relief, particularly for arthritis. The active compound in willow bark is salicin, which is chemically similar to aspirin and possesses anti-inflammatory, analgesic, and antipyretic properties.

Ingredients:

- 1-2 teaspoons of dried willow bark (Salix alba)
- 2 cups of water
- Honey or lemon (optional, for taste)

Instructions:

1. **Measure the Willow Bark:** Begin by measuring 1-2 teaspoons of dried willow bark. The amount can be adjusted based on the severity of pain and individual tolerance.
2. **Boil Water:** Bring 2 cups of water to a boil in a small saucepan.
3. **Add Willow Bark:** Once the water reaches a rolling boil, add the dried willow bark.
4. **Simmer:** Reduce the heat and let the mixture simmer for about 10-15 minutes. This slow simmering process helps to extract the active compounds from the willow bark.
5. **Strain:** After simmering, remove the saucepan from heat and strain the decoction through a fine mesh strainer or cheesecloth into a cup or teapot.
6. **Add Flavor (Optional):** If desired, add honey or lemon to enhance the taste.
7. **Serve:** The decoction is ready to be consumed.

Dosage:

- It is recommended to drink 1 cup of willow bark decoction up to three times a day.
- Due to the presence of salicin, it's important to consult with a healthcare provider before regular use, especially for individuals who are sensitive to aspirin, pregnant, breastfeeding, or taking other medications.

The Role of Willow Bark as a Natural Pain Reliever

Historical Context and Mechanism of Action: Willow bark has a long history of use in traditional medicine. Ancient civilizations, including the Egyptians and Native Americans, used willow bark to alleviate pain and reduce fever. The primary active compound, salicin, is metabolized in the body to produce salicylic acid, which inhibits the production of prostaglandins, compounds that cause inflammation, pain, and fever. By reducing prostaglandin production, willow bark effectively diminishes pain and inflammation, making it a valuable natural remedy for arthritis.

Scientific Evidence: Modern scientific studies support the use of willow bark for pain relief. Research has shown that willow bark can be as effective as non-steroidal anti-inflammatory drugs (NSAIDs) like aspirin and ibuprofen but with fewer side effects. One study published in the journal *Phytotherapy Research* found that patients with osteoarthritis experienced significant pain reduction after taking willow bark extract. Another study in the *American Journal of Medicine* confirmed its efficacy in reducing lower back pain.

Benefits for Arthritis: Arthritis is characterized by joint inflammation, stiffness, and pain. Willow bark's anti-inflammatory properties help reduce the swelling and discomfort associated with arthritis. Regular consumption of willow bark decoction can lead to improved joint mobility and decreased pain, enhancing the quality of life for arthritis sufferers.

Safety and Precautions: While willow bark is generally safe for most people, it is essential to use it cautiously. Overconsumption can lead to side effects such as stomach upset, ulcers, and bleeding disorders due to its salicin content. Individuals with allergies to aspirin or NSAIDs should avoid willow bark. Additionally, it should not be given to children due to the risk of Reye's syndrome, a rare but serious condition.

Green Tea and Ginger Infusion

Recipe: Green Tea with Fresh Ginger

Green tea and ginger are both renowned for their health benefits, particularly their anti-inflammatory and antioxidant properties. When combined, they create a powerful infusion that can help manage arthritis symptoms by reducing inflammation and oxidative stress in the body.

Ingredients:

- 1 green tea bag or 1 teaspoon of loose green tea leaves
- 1-inch piece of fresh ginger root
- 2 cups of water
- Honey or lemon (optional, for taste)

Instructions:

1. **Prepare the Ginger:** Peel and slice the fresh ginger root into thin pieces.
2. **Boil Water:** Bring 2 cups of water to a boil in a saucepan.
3. **Add Ginger:** Once the water is boiling, add the ginger slices and let them simmer for about 5 minutes.
4. **Add Green Tea:** After simmering the ginger, add the green tea bag or loose green tea leaves to the saucepan.

5. **Steep:** Remove the saucepan from heat and let the mixture steep for 3-5 minutes. This allows the green tea to infuse with the ginger.
6. **Strain:** Strain the infusion into a cup using a fine mesh strainer or tea infuser.
7. **Add Flavor (Optional):** Add honey or lemon if desired.
8. **Serve:** The infusion is ready to be enjoyed.

Dosage:

- It is recommended to drink 1-2 cups of green tea with fresh ginger daily. For optimal benefits, consume the infusion in the morning or early afternoon.

Anti-Inflammatory Properties of Green Tea and Ginger

Green Tea: Green tea is rich in polyphenols, particularly catechins like epigallocatechin gallate (EGCG), which have potent antioxidant and anti-inflammatory effects. These compounds help to neutralize free radicals and reduce inflammation in the body, making green tea beneficial for managing arthritis symptoms.

Scientific Evidence: Studies have shown that EGCG can inhibit the production of inflammatory cytokines and enzymes involved in arthritis. A study published in the journal *Arthritis Research & Therapy* demonstrated that EGCG could reduce joint damage and inflammation in animal models of rheumatoid arthritis. Additionally, green tea's antioxidant properties help protect cartilage and joint tissues from oxidative stress, which is crucial for arthritis management.

Ginger: Ginger contains bioactive compounds such as gingerol and shogaol, which have strong anti-inflammatory and analgesic properties. These compounds inhibit the production of pro-inflammatory cytokines and enzymes, reducing inflammation and pain associated with arthritis.

Scientific Evidence: A study published in the journal *Osteoarthritis and Cartilage* found that ginger extract significantly reduced pain and stiffness in patients with osteoarthritis.

Another study in *The Journal of Medicinal Food* reported that ginger could decrease markers of inflammation in people with rheumatoid arthritis.

Combined Benefits: The combination of green tea and ginger creates a synergistic effect, enhancing their individual benefits. Together, they help to reduce inflammation, alleviate pain, and improve joint function in arthritis patients. Regular consumption of this infusion can lead to long-term improvements in arthritis symptoms and overall joint health.

Safety and Precautions: Green tea and ginger are generally safe for most people. However, excessive consumption of green tea can lead to side effects such as insomnia, stomach upset, and headaches due to its caffeine content. Ginger, when consumed in large amounts, can cause digestive issues such as heartburn and diarrhea. It is important to consume these ingredients in moderation and consult with a healthcare provider if you have any underlying health conditions or are taking medications.

By incorporating willow bark decoction and green tea with ginger infusion into your daily routine, you can harness the natural healing properties of these ingredients to manage arthritis symptoms effectively. These remedies offer a holistic approach to arthritis care, supporting pain relief, reducing inflammation, and promoting overall joint health.

CHAPTER 4

Integrating Herbal Remedies into Your Daily Routine

Tips for Consistency

Integrating herbal remedies into your daily routine is essential for managing high cholesterol effectively. Consistency in herbal treatment can significantly impact your cholesterol levels and overall cardiovascular health. Here's how to incorporate these remedies seamlessly into your life:

1. **Start with Small, Manageable Changes:** Begin by incorporating one or two herbal remedies into your daily routine. For example, start with a morning cup of green tea or a daily spoonful of flaxseed. Gradually add more herbs as you become accustomed to your new routine.

2. **Set Specific Goals:** Define clear, achievable goals for your herbal regimen. For instance, you might aim to consume a specific amount of a particular herb each day. Setting goals helps track progress and keeps you motivated.

3. **Create a Schedule:** Establish a daily schedule that includes time for preparing and consuming your herbal remedies. Consistency is key, so choose times that fit well with your existing routines, such as having herbal tea with breakfast or adding flaxseed to your lunch.

4. **Keep a Herbal Journal:** Maintain a journal to track the herbs you are using, the dosage, and any effects you notice. Documenting your experience helps you monitor progress and make adjustments if needed.

5. **Use Reminders:** Set reminders on your phone or calendar to ensure you don't forget to take your herbs. This can be especially helpful when starting a new regimen or when incorporating multiple herbs.

6. **Incorporate Herbs into Meals:** Adding herbs to your meals can make them more enjoyable and ensure you get your daily dose. For example, use turmeric in your cooking or add herbs like garlic to your dishes.

7. **Seek Support:** Share your herbal regimen with family or friends who can offer encouragement and hold you accountable. You might also consider joining a support group or online community focused on herbal health.

Creating a Personalized Herbal Plan

A personalized herbal plan tailored to your specific needs can maximize the benefits of herbal remedies for managing high cholesterol. Here's how to create an effective plan:

1. **Assess Your Health Needs:** Begin by evaluating your current health status, including your cholesterol levels and any other relevant health conditions. Consult with a healthcare professional to get a clear understanding of your needs.

2. **Choose Appropriate Herbs:** Select herbs known for their cholesterol-lowering properties. Some effective herbs include:

   o **Garlic:** Known to reduce LDL cholesterol and increase HDL cholesterol.

   o **Flaxseed:** Rich in omega-3 fatty acids and fiber, which help lower cholesterol.

   o **Psyllium:** A soluble fiber that helps reduce LDL cholesterol levels.

   o **Turmeric:** Contains curcumin, which may help reduce cholesterol levels.

3. **Determine Dosage:** Based on your chosen herbs, establish the appropriate dosage. Follow the recommended dosages provided for each herb to ensure effectiveness and avoid adverse effects.

4. **Plan Your Daily Routine:** Create a daily schedule that integrates your herbal remedies. For example:

- Morning: Take a flaxseed supplement or add ground flaxseed to your breakfast.

- Afternoon: Drink a cup of garlic tea or add garlic to your lunch.

- Evening: Incorporate turmeric into your dinner or take a turmeric supplement.

5. **Monitor and Adjust:** Regularly monitor your cholesterol levels and overall health. Adjust your herbal plan as needed based on your progress and any feedback from your healthcare provider.

6. **Stay Informed:** Keep yourself updated on new research and developments related to herbal remedies and cholesterol management. This knowledge will help you make informed decisions and adjustments to your plan.

Chapter 5: Lifestyle Changes for Managing High Cholesterol

Exercise and Physical Activity

Regular physical activity is crucial for managing high cholesterol. Exercise helps improve your overall cardiovascular health and can lead to significant reductions in cholesterol levels. Here's how to incorporate exercise into your lifestyle:

1. **Understand the Benefits:** Exercise helps increase HDL (good) cholesterol while lowering LDL (bad) cholesterol and triglycerides. It also aids in weight management and reduces the risk of cardiovascular diseases.

2. **Choose Activities You Enjoy:** Select exercises that you find enjoyable and can sustain long-term. Activities such as walking, jogging, swimming, cycling, and dancing can be both fun and effective.

3. **Aim for Consistency:** Strive for at least 150 minutes of moderate-intensity exercise per week or 75 minutes of vigorous-intensity exercise. Break this into manageable sessions, such as 30 minutes a day, five times a week.

4. **Incorporate Strength Training:** Include strength training exercises at least twice a week. Activities like weightlifting or body-weight exercises help build muscle mass, which can further enhance cholesterol levels.

5. **Stay Active Throughout the Day:** Find opportunities to stay active beyond your scheduled exercise sessions. Take the stairs instead of the elevator, walk or bike for short trips, and incorporate physical activity into your daily routine.

6. **Set Realistic Goals:** Set achievable fitness goals that motivate you to stay active. Track your progress and celebrate milestones, such as completing a certain number of workouts or achieving personal fitness goals.

7. **Combine Exercise with a Healthy Diet:** Pair your exercise routine with a balanced diet rich in fruits, vegetables, whole grains, and lean proteins. Combining diet and exercise enhances the effectiveness of cholesterol management.

Stress Management Techniques

Chronic stress can negatively impact cholesterol levels and overall heart health. Managing stress effectively is essential for maintaining healthy cholesterol levels. Here's how to incorporate stress management techniques into your lifestyle:

1. **Identify Stress Triggers:** Recognize the sources of stress in your life. Understanding what triggers stress can help you address these factors and implement coping strategies.

2. **Practice Mindfulness and Meditation:** Mindfulness and meditation techniques can help reduce stress and improve emotional well-being. Incorporate practices such as deep breathing exercises, guided meditation, or yoga into your daily routine.

3. **Engage in Relaxing Activities:** Find activities that help you relax and unwind. This could include hobbies, reading, spending time in nature, or listening to calming music. Engaging in these activities regularly can lower stress levels.

4. **Maintain a Healthy Work-Life Balance:** Strive for a balanced approach to work and personal life. Set boundaries to prevent work from overwhelming your personal time and ensure you have time to relax and recharge.

5. **Get Adequate Sleep:** Prioritize quality sleep, as poor sleep can contribute to stress and negatively affect cholesterol levels. Aim for 7-9 hours of restful sleep each night.

6. **Seek Social Support:** Build a support network of friends, family, or support groups. Social connections provide emotional support and help reduce stress levels.

7. **Consider Professional Help:** If stress becomes overwhelming or difficult to manage on your own, consider seeking help from a mental health professional. Therapy or counseling can provide valuable strategies for coping with stress.

8. **Practice Gratitude:** Cultivating a sense of gratitude can shift your focus away from stressors and improve your overall mood. Regularly reflect on the positive aspects of your life and express appreciation for them.

By integrating these strategies into your daily routine, you can effectively manage high cholesterol and improve your overall cardiovascular health. Combining herbal remedies with lifestyle changes creates a comprehensive approach to cholesterol management.

CHAPTER 6

Dr. Barbara O'Neill Cure for Arthritis

Dr. Barbara O'Neill is a renowned natural health practitioner known for her holistic approach to health and wellness. Her teachings emphasize the use of natural remedies and lifestyle changes to manage and cure various health conditions, including arthritis. Arthritis is a term often used to refer to joint pain or joint disease and encompasses over 100 different types of conditions. The most common forms are osteoarthritis (OA) and rheumatoid arthritis (RA).

Arthritis can cause debilitating pain, stiffness, swelling, and decreased range of motion in the affected joints. These symptoms can worsen over time, leading to severe discomfort and a diminished quality of life. Traditional treatments for arthritis typically involve medications to manage pain and inflammation, but these can come with significant side effects. Dr. Barbara O'Neill advocates for a natural approach that focuses on diet, exercise, and herbal remedies to alleviate arthritis symptoms and improve overall joint health.

In this comprehensive guide, we will explore several natural remedies recommended by Dr. Barbara O'Neill for managing arthritis. These remedies include the use of cayenne pepper and olive oil salve, as well as ginger and garlic soup, both known for their potent anti-inflammatory and analgesic properties.

Cayenne Pepper and Olive Oil Salve

Recipe: Cayenne Pepper and Olive Oil Pain Relief Salve

Ingredients:

- 1/2 cup of olive oil

- 2 tablespoons of cayenne pepper powder

- 1/4 cup of beeswax pellets

- 10 drops of peppermint essential oil (optional)

Instructions:

1. In a double boiler, gently heat the olive oil over low heat.

2. Add the cayenne pepper powder to the oil and stir well to combine.

3. Allow the mixture to infuse on low heat for about 30 minutes, stirring occasionally.

4. After 30 minutes, strain the oil through a cheesecloth or fine mesh strainer to remove the cayenne pepper solids.

5. Return the infused oil to the double boiler and add the beeswax pellets.

6. Stir continuously until the beeswax is completely melted and the mixture is smooth.

7. Remove from heat and add the peppermint essential oil, if using. Stir well to combine.

8. Pour the mixture into a glass jar or tin and allow it to cool and solidify.

Dosage and How to Use:

- Apply a small amount of the salve to the affected joints 2-3 times a day.

- Gently massage the salve into the skin until fully absorbed.

- Wash hands thoroughly after application to avoid transferring the salve to sensitive areas such as the eyes or mucous membranes.

The Analgesic Properties of Cayenne Pepper

Cayenne pepper contains a compound called capsaicin, which is responsible for its heat and analgesic properties. Capsaicin works by depleting a neurotransmitter called substance P, which is involved in transmitting pain signals to the brain. By reducing the levels of substance P, capsaicin can effectively diminish the sensation of pain.

Studies have shown that topical application of capsaicin can significantly reduce pain in people with arthritis. Capsaicin creams and salves are particularly effective for osteoarthritis and rheumatoid arthritis. The warmth generated by the cayenne pepper can also help to relax muscles and improve blood flow to the affected area, further aiding in pain relief and promoting healing.

Olive oil, the base for this salve, is rich in antioxidants and has anti-inflammatory properties of its own. It helps to nourish and moisturize the skin, making it an ideal carrier oil for the cayenne pepper. Together, these ingredients create a potent natural remedy for managing arthritis pain.

Ginger and Garlic Anti-Inflammatory Soup

Recipe: Ginger and Garlic Soup

Ingredients:

- 1 tablespoon of olive oil

- 1 medium onion, chopped

- 3 cloves of garlic, minced

- 1 tablespoon of fresh ginger, grated

- 4 cups of vegetable broth

- 2 carrots, sliced

- 2 celery stalks, sliced

- 1 cup of chopped spinach or kale

- Salt and pepper to taste

- Fresh lemon juice (optional)

Instructions:

1. Heat the olive oil in a large pot over medium heat.

2. Add the chopped onion and sauté until it becomes translucent, about 5 minutes.

3. Add the minced garlic and grated ginger, and sauté for another 2-3 minutes until fragrant.

4. Pour in the vegetable broth and bring to a boil.

5. Add the sliced carrots and celery, and reduce the heat to a simmer.

6. Cook until the vegetables are tender, about 15-20 minutes.

7. Stir in the chopped spinach or kale and cook for an additional 5 minutes.

8. Season with salt and pepper to taste.

9. For an extra burst of flavor, add a squeeze of fresh lemon juice before serving.

Dosage and How to Use:

- Consume one bowl of ginger and garlic soup daily.

- For best results, include this soup as a regular part of your diet, aiming to have it at least 3-4 times a week.

Combining Ginger and Garlic for Arthritis Relief

Ginger and garlic are two powerful natural anti-inflammatory agents that have been used for centuries in traditional medicine. Both of these ingredients contain compounds that can help reduce inflammation and pain, making them highly effective for managing arthritis symptoms.

Ginger: Ginger contains bioactive compounds like gingerol, which have potent anti-inflammatory and antioxidant effects. Gingerol has been shown to inhibit the production of inflammatory cytokines and enzymes, which play a key role in the inflammatory process associated with arthritis. Regular consumption of ginger can help reduce joint pain and improve mobility in individuals with arthritis. In addition to its anti-inflammatory properties, ginger also has analgesic effects, helping to relieve pain naturally.

Garlic: Garlic is rich in sulfur compounds, such as allicin, which have been shown to have anti-inflammatory and immune-boosting properties. Allicin and other sulfur compounds in garlic can help reduce the production of pro-inflammatory cytokines and modulate the immune response, making garlic particularly beneficial for individuals with autoimmune forms of arthritis, like rheumatoid arthritis. Garlic also has antioxidant properties, which can help protect the joints from oxidative stress and further damage.

Synergistic Effects: When combined, ginger and garlic create a synergistic effect that enhances their individual anti-inflammatory and analgesic properties. This combination can help to reduce inflammation more effectively, alleviate pain, and improve overall joint function. The ginger and garlic soup recipe provided is an excellent way to incorporate these powerful ingredients into your diet and take advantage of their combined benefits.

By following Dr. Barbara O'Neill's natural approach to arthritis management, incorporating remedies like the cayenne pepper and olive oil salve, as well as the ginger and garlic anti-inflammatory soup, you can effectively reduce inflammation, alleviate pain, and improve your quality of life. Remember, consistency is key, and it's important to make these remedies a regular part of your routine for the best results. Always consult with a healthcare professional before making any significant changes to your treatment plan, especially if you are currently taking medications for arthritis.

CHAPTER 7

Dr. Barbara O'Neill Cure for Arthritis: Turmeric and Ginger Anti-Inflammatory Blend

Introduction

Arthritis is a common condition characterized by inflammation and pain in the joints. Conventional treatments often include medications that can have side effects. Dr. Barbara O'Neill's natural approach offers a holistic way to manage and potentially alleviate arthritis symptoms using natural remedies. One of the most effective natural remedies for arthritis is the **Turmeric and Ginger Anti-Inflammatory Blend**.

Turmeric and Ginger: Nature's Anti-Inflammatories

Turmeric and ginger are renowned for their powerful anti-inflammatory properties. Turmeric contains curcumin, a compound with strong anti-inflammatory and antioxidant effects. Ginger, on the other hand, has gingerol, which helps reduce inflammation and pain.

Benefits of Turmeric for Arthritis

- **Anti-Inflammatory Properties**: Curcumin in turmeric inhibits molecules that play a role in inflammation.

- **Antioxidant Effects**: Helps protect cells from damage caused by free radicals.

- **Pain Relief**: Can help reduce the pain associated with arthritis.

Benefits of Ginger for Arthritis

- **Reduction of Inflammatory Markers**: Gingerol reduces the production of cytokines and chemokines, which are involved in the inflammatory response.

- **Pain Management**: Ginger helps alleviate the pain linked to arthritis.

- **Improved Joint Function**: Regular consumption can lead to better joint mobility and function.

Ingredients

- 1 teaspoon ground turmeric

- 1 teaspoon ground ginger

- 1 cup of warm water

- 1 tablespoon honey (optional)

- 1 tablespoon lemon juice (optional)

Instructions

1. **Combine Turmeric and Ginger**: Mix the ground turmeric and ginger in a cup.

2. **Add Warm Water**: Pour the warm water over the mixture and stir well.

3. **Sweeten**: Add honey and lemon juice if desired for taste.

4. **Stir and Drink**: Stir thoroughly and drink immediately.

Dosage and How to Use

- **Dosage**: Drink one cup of this blend twice daily.

- **How to Use**: Consume in the morning on an empty stomach and again in the evening. Consistent use over several weeks is necessary to observe significant improvements in arthritis symptoms.

Flaxseed and Chia Seed Pudding

Introduction

Flaxseeds and chia seeds are excellent sources of omega-3 fatty acids, which are essential for reducing inflammation and improving joint health. These seeds also contain high levels of fiber, antioxidants, and other nutrients that support overall health.

- **Anti-Inflammatory Effects**: Omega-3s reduce the production of inflammatory molecules.

- **Joint Lubrication**: Helps keep joints well-lubricated, reducing stiffness and pain.

- **Bone Health**: Supports bone density and strength, important for arthritis sufferers.

Recipe: Flaxseed and Chia Seed Anti-Inflammatory Pudding

Ingredients

- 2 tablespoons chia seeds

- 1 tablespoon ground flaxseed

- 1 cup almond milk (or any plant-based milk)

- 1 teaspoon vanilla extract

- 1 tablespoon honey or maple syrup

- Fresh fruits or nuts for topping (optional)

Instructions

1. **Combine Ingredients**: In a bowl, mix the chia seeds, ground flaxseed, almond milk, vanilla extract, and honey or maple syrup.

2. **Stir Well**: Ensure the seeds are evenly distributed in the liquid.

3. **Refrigerate**: Cover the bowl and refrigerate for at least 4 hours or overnight.

4. **Serve**: Stir again before serving and top with fresh fruits or nuts if desired.

Dosage and How to Use

- **Dosage**: Consume one serving (about half a cup) daily.

- **How to Use**: Eat the pudding as a breakfast option or a snack. Regular intake supports reduced inflammation and improved joint health.

Dandelion Greens Salad

Introduction

Dandelion greens are a powerful detoxifying and anti-inflammatory food. They are rich in vitamins A, C, and K, as well as minerals like calcium and iron. Dandelion greens also have diuretic properties, which help reduce joint swelling and pain associated with arthritis.

Detoxifying and Anti-Inflammatory Benefits of Dandelion Greens

- **Detoxification**: Supports liver function and aids in the elimination of toxins that can contribute to inflammation.

- **Anti-Inflammatory Properties**: Contains phytonutrients that reduce inflammation.

- **Nutrient-Dense**: Provides essential vitamins and minerals that support overall joint health and reduce arthritis symptoms.

Recipe: Fresh Dandelion Greens Salad

Ingredients

- 2 cups fresh dandelion greens, washed and chopped

- 1 avocado, sliced

- 1/2 cup cherry tomatoes, halved

- 1/4 cup red onion, thinly sliced

- 1/4 cup crumbled feta cheese (optional)

- 2 tablespoons olive oil

- 1 tablespoon lemon juice

- Salt and pepper to taste

Instructions

1. **Prepare Greens**: Place the washed and chopped dandelion greens in a large salad bowl.

2. **Add Vegetables**: Add the sliced avocado, cherry tomatoes, and red onion to the bowl.

3. **Add Cheese**: Sprinkle the crumbled feta cheese over the salad if using.

4. **Dress Salad**: In a small bowl, whisk together the olive oil, lemon juice, salt, and pepper.

5. **Toss and Serve**: Pour the dressing over the salad and toss well to combine. Serve immediately.

Dosage and How to Use

- **Dosage**: Consume one serving (about one cup) of the salad daily.

- **How to Use**: Eat the salad as a side dish with your main meal or as a light lunch. Regular consumption aids in detoxification and reduces inflammation, contributing to overall joint health and alleviation of arthritis symptoms.

Dr. Barbara O'Neill's approach to curing arthritis emphasizes natural remedies that target inflammation and support joint health. The **Turmeric and Ginger Anti-Inflammatory Blend, Flaxseed and Chia Seed Anti-Inflammatory Pudding**, and **Fresh Dandelion Greens Salad** are three potent recipes that provide a holistic and effective way to manage arthritis symptoms. Incorporating these natural remedies into your daily routine can lead to significant improvements in joint function, reduced pain, and enhanced overall well-being.

CHAPTER 7

Arthritis is a debilitating condition that affects millions of people worldwide. It causes inflammation, pain, and stiffness in the joints, which can significantly impact one's quality of life. Dr. Barbara O'Neill, a renowned naturopath, has explored various natural remedies to alleviate the symptoms of arthritis. Among these, herbal treatments have shown considerable promise. This section will delve into three specific remedies: Willow Bark Decoction, Rosemary and Thyme Infused Oil, and Parsley and Celery Juice.

Willow Bark Decoction

Introduction: Willow bark has been used for centuries to treat pain and inflammation. It contains salicin, a compound similar to aspirin, which makes it an effective natural remedy for arthritis.

Ingredients:

- 2 tablespoons of dried willow bark

- 2 cups of water

Preparation:

1. Add the dried willow bark to the water in a saucepan.

2. Bring the mixture to a boil.

3. Reduce the heat and let it simmer for about 10-15 minutes.

4. Remove from heat and strain the liquid to remove the bark.

5. Allow the decoction to cool before drinking.

Dosage and Usage:

- Drink one cup of willow bark decoction twice daily, preferably in the morning and evening.

- It can be consumed warm or at room temperature.

- It is advisable to consult a healthcare professional before starting this remedy, especially if you are on other medications.

Benefits:

- **Anti-inflammatory Properties:** Willow bark is known for its anti-inflammatory effects, which can help reduce joint inflammation.

- **Pain Relief:** The salicin in willow bark works similarly to aspirin, providing pain relief without the synthetic chemicals found in over-the-counter medications.

- **Natural Origin:** Being a natural remedy, it has fewer side effects compared to conventional drugs.

Precautions:

- Do not use if allergic to aspirin.

- Avoid during pregnancy or breastfeeding.

- Consult with a healthcare provider if you have any pre-existing medical conditions.

Rosemary and Thyme Infused Oil

Introduction: Rosemary and thyme are herbs with potent anti-inflammatory and analgesic properties. When infused in oil, they can be used for massage to alleviate arthritis symptoms.

Recipe: Rosemary and Thyme Infused Olive Oil

Ingredients:

- 1 cup of extra virgin olive oil

- 2 tablespoons of dried rosemary

- 2 tablespoons of dried thyme

Preparation:

1. Pour the olive oil into a small saucepan and heat gently.

2. Add the dried rosemary and thyme to the oil.

3. Allow the mixture to simmer on low heat for about 30 minutes, ensuring the oil does not boil.

4. Remove from heat and let it cool.

5. Strain the oil to remove the herbs.

6. Store the infused oil in a dark glass bottle away from direct sunlight.

Dosage and Usage:

- Use the infused oil for massage once or twice daily.

- Apply a small amount of oil to the affected joints and massage gently in circular motions for about 10-15 minutes.

- For best results, use after a warm bath to enhance absorption.

Benefits:

- **Anti-inflammatory Effects:** Both rosemary and thyme have compounds that reduce inflammation, helping to alleviate pain and swelling in the joints.

- **Improved Circulation:** Massaging with this oil can improve blood flow to the affected areas, promoting healing.

- **Relaxation:** The aroma of rosemary and thyme can also help in relaxing the mind and body, reducing the overall discomfort associated with arthritis.

Precautions:

- Conduct a patch test to ensure there is no allergic reaction to the oil.

- Do not use on broken or irritated skin.

- Consult a healthcare professional if you are pregnant, breastfeeding, or have a medical condition.

Parsley and Celery Juice

Introduction: Parsley and celery are rich in anti-inflammatory compounds and essential nutrients that can help manage arthritis symptoms. Juicing these vegetables allows for easy consumption and quick absorption of their beneficial properties.

Recipe: Parsley and Celery Juice

Ingredients:

- 1 cup of fresh parsley leaves

- 3-4 celery stalks

- 1 cucumber (optional, for added hydration)

- 1 lemon (optional, for flavor)

- 1 cup of water

Preparation:

1. Wash all the ingredients thoroughly.

2. Chop the parsley and celery into smaller pieces.

3. If using, peel and chop the cucumber.

4. Add all the ingredients to a blender, including the water.

5. Blend until smooth.

6. Strain the mixture using a fine mesh sieve or cheesecloth to remove the pulp.

7. Squeeze the lemon juice into the strained liquid (optional).

8. Serve immediately for the best nutrient retention.

Dosage and Usage:

- Drink one glass of parsley and celery juice once daily, preferably in the morning on an empty stomach.

- For optimal benefits, consume fresh juice immediately after preparation.

Benefits:

- **Anti-inflammatory Benefits:** Both parsley and celery contain antioxidants and anti-inflammatory compounds like apigenin and luteolin, which help reduce inflammation in the joints.

- **Detoxification:** Parsley is known for its diuretic properties, helping to flush out toxins from the body that may contribute to inflammation.

- **Nutrient-Rich:** This juice provides essential vitamins and minerals like Vitamin C, Vitamin K, and potassium, which are crucial for joint health.

Precautions:

- People with kidney issues should consult their doctor before consuming large amounts of parsley.

- If you experience any adverse reactions, discontinue use and consult a healthcare professional.

Juicing for Anti-Inflammatory Benefits

Juicing is an excellent way to incorporate anti-inflammatory foods into your diet. Fresh juices made from vegetables and herbs like parsley and celery provide concentrated doses of vitamins, minerals, and antioxidants that help combat inflammation.

Why Juicing Works:

- **Concentration of Nutrients:** Juicing extracts the liquid from fruits and vegetables, leaving behind most of the fiber but concentrating the vitamins, minerals, and phytonutrients.

- **Ease of Digestion:** The nutrients in juice are easily absorbed by the body, allowing for quicker and more efficient nutrient uptake.

- **Hydration:** Juices provide hydration, which is essential for maintaining joint health and reducing inflammation.

Best Practices for Juicing:

- **Use Fresh Ingredients:** Always use fresh, organic produce to ensure maximum nutrient content and avoid pesticides.

- **Consume Immediately:** Drink juice immediately after preparation to prevent nutrient degradation.

- **Balanced Diet:** Use juicing as a supplement to a balanced diet, not as a replacement for whole fruits and vegetables.

Conclusion: Incorporating natural remedies such as Willow Bark Decoction, Rosemary and Thyme Infused Oil, and Parsley and Celery Juice can significantly aid in managing arthritis symptoms. These treatments, backed by Dr. Barbara O'Neill's expertise, offer natural, effective, and holistic approaches to reducing pain and inflammation associated with arthritis. Always consult with a healthcare professional before starting any new treatment regimen, especially if you have underlying health conditions or are taking other medications.

CHAPTER 7

Fenugreek Seed Tea

Fenugreek (Trigonella foenum-graecum) is a powerful herb that has been used for centuries in traditional medicine for its numerous health benefits. One of the most notable uses of fenugreek seeds is their potential to lower high cholesterol levels. Fenugreek seeds contain saponins, which are compounds that help reduce the body's absorption of cholesterol. They also contain fiber, which can bind to cholesterol in the digestive system and help remove it from the body.

Recipe: Fenugreek Seed Tea

Ingredients:

- 1 teaspoon fenugreek seeds

- 1 cup of water

- Honey or lemon (optional, for taste)

Instructions:

1. Boil the water in a small pot.

2. Add the fenugreek seeds to the boiling water.

3. Reduce the heat and let it simmer for about 5 minutes.

4. Remove from heat and let it steep for another 5 minutes.

5. Strain the tea into a cup.

6. Add honey or lemon if desired for taste.

Dosage: Drink one cup of fenugreek seed tea twice daily, preferably in the morning and evening, to help manage high cholesterol levels. It is important to note that consistency is key, and regular consumption over a period of several weeks is necessary to observe significant effects.

Fenugreek Seeds for Reducing Arthritis Swelling

Beyond cholesterol management, fenugreek seeds are also beneficial for reducing inflammation and swelling associated with arthritis. The seeds contain anti-inflammatory properties that can help alleviate joint pain and swelling.

Recipe: Fenugreek Seed Tea for Arthritis

Ingredients:

- 1 teaspoon fenugreek seeds

- 1 cup of water

- Honey or lemon (optional, for taste)

Instructions:

1. Boil the water in a small pot.

2. Add the fenugreek seeds to the boiling water.

3. Reduce the heat and let it simmer for about 5 minutes.

4. Remove from heat and let it steep for another 5 minutes.

5. Strain the tea into a cup.

6. Add honey or lemon if desired for taste.

Dosage: Drink one cup of fenugreek seed tea twice daily. This can be taken alongside other treatments for arthritis as part of a comprehensive approach to managing symptoms.

Chamomile and Lavender Relaxation Tea

Chamomile (Matricaria chamomilla) and lavender (Lavandula angustifolia) are two well-known herbs famous for their calming and relaxing properties. These herbs can be combined to create a soothing tea that helps reduce stress and promote relaxation. Moreover, reducing stress is beneficial for overall heart health, including managing high cholesterol levels, as stress can contribute to elevated cholesterol.

Recipe: Chamomile and Lavender Tea

Ingredients:

- 1 teaspoon dried chamomile flowers

- 1 teaspoon dried lavender flowers

- 1 cup of water

- Honey (optional, for taste)

Instructions:

1. Boil the water in a small pot.

2. Add the chamomile and lavender flowers to the boiling water.

3. Reduce the heat and let it simmer for about 5 minutes.

4. Remove from heat and let it steep for another 5 minutes.

5. Strain the tea into a cup.

6. Add honey if desired for taste.

Dosage: Drink one cup of chamomile and lavender tea in the evening before bedtime. This can help promote relaxation and improve sleep quality, which is essential for overall health and well-being.

Relaxation and Pain Relief Through Herbal Teas

Herbal teas, such as chamomile and lavender tea, are effective natural remedies for relaxation and pain relief. Regular consumption of these teas can help alleviate symptoms of anxiety, stress, and chronic pain, which are often associated with various health conditions, including high cholesterol.

Chamomile and Lavender Tea for Pain Relief

Ingredients:

- 1 teaspoon dried chamomile flowers

- 1 teaspoon dried lavender flowers

- 1 cup of water

- Honey (optional, for taste)

Instructions:

1. Boil the water in a small pot.

2. Add the chamomile and lavender flowers to the boiling water.

3. Reduce the heat and let it simmer for about 5 minutes.

4. Remove from heat and let it steep for another 5 minutes.

5. Strain the tea into a cup.

6. Add honey if desired for taste.

Dosage: Drink one cup of chamomile and lavender tea up to three times daily to help manage pain and stress. The anti-inflammatory properties of chamomile and the soothing effects of lavender can work together to provide relief from various types of pain, including headaches and muscle tension.

Health Benefits and Mechanisms of Action

Fenugreek Seeds:

- **Cholesterol Management:** Fenugreek seeds are rich in soluble fiber, which can help lower cholesterol levels. The saponins in fenugreek seeds also reduce the absorption of cholesterol in the intestines.

- **Anti-Inflammatory Properties:** Fenugreek seeds contain compounds that have anti-inflammatory effects, which can help reduce pain and swelling in conditions like arthritis.

Chamomile and Lavender:

- **Relaxation and Stress Reduction:** Both chamomile and lavender have been shown to have calming effects on the nervous system, helping to reduce stress and promote relaxation.

- **Pain Relief:** Chamomile has anti-inflammatory and analgesic properties, making it useful for pain relief. Lavender also has mild pain-relieving properties and can help alleviate headaches and muscle tension.

Integrating Herbal Teas into a Cholesterol-Lowering Regimen

Incorporating fenugreek seed tea and chamomile and lavender tea into a daily routine can be an effective part of a comprehensive approach to managing high cholesterol. Here are some additional tips:

1. **Balanced Diet:** Alongside herbal teas, maintain a diet rich in fruits, vegetables, whole grains, and lean proteins. Foods high in fiber, such as oats and barley, can also help lower cholesterol levels.

2. **Regular Exercise:** Engage in regular physical activity, such as brisk walking, swimming, or cycling, to improve cardiovascular health and help manage cholesterol levels.

3. **Stress Management:** Practice stress-reducing techniques such as yoga, meditation, and deep breathing exercises. Herbal teas like chamomile and lavender can complement these practices.

4. **Hydration:** Stay well-hydrated by drinking plenty of water throughout the day. Herbal teas can be a part of your hydration routine.

5. **Consistency:** Regular and consistent consumption of herbal teas is key to observing their benefits. Aim to make these teas a part of your daily routine.

Precautions and Considerations

While herbal teas can be beneficial, it is important to consider the following precautions:

- **Consultation with Healthcare Provider:** Before starting any new herbal regimen, especially if you have existing health conditions or are taking medications, consult with your healthcare provider.

- **Allergies:** Ensure that you are not allergic to any of the ingredients used in the teas.

- **Moderation:** While herbal teas are generally safe, excessive consumption can lead to adverse effects. Stick to the recommended dosages.

- **Pregnancy and Nursing:** Pregnant and nursing women should consult with their healthcare provider before consuming herbal teas.

Conclusion

Fenugreek seed tea and chamomile and lavender tea offer a range of health benefits, particularly for managing high cholesterol and reducing stress and pain. By incorporating these herbal teas into your daily routine, alongside a balanced diet and regular exercise, you can support your overall cardiovascular health and well-being. Remember to consult with a healthcare provider to ensure that these remedies are appropriate for your individual health needs.

CHAPTER 8

Dr. Barbara O'Neill Cure for Arthritis: Turmeric and Black Pepper Capsules

Arthritis is a common condition characterized by inflammation of the joints, leading to pain, stiffness, and reduced mobility. It can affect people of all ages, but is more prevalent among the elderly. Managing arthritis often involves addressing inflammation, pain, and joint damage. Natural remedies, particularly those that harness the power of anti-inflammatory herbs like turmeric, have been advocated by many health experts, including Dr. Barbara O'Neill.

Turmeric, a golden-yellow spice derived from the root of the *Curcuma longa* plant, has long been used in traditional medicine for its potent anti-inflammatory and antioxidant properties. The active compound in turmeric, curcumin, is known to inhibit the activity of enzymes and cytokines that promote inflammation. However, curcumin's bioavailability—the extent to which it is absorbed and utilized by the body—is relatively low. This is where black pepper comes into play. Black pepper contains piperine, a compound that enhances the absorption of curcumin by up to 2,000%.

Combining turmeric with black pepper in capsule form provides a convenient and effective way to deliver these compounds to the body, making it a popular natural remedy for managing arthritis symptoms.

Recipe: Homemade Turmeric and Black Pepper Capsules

Ingredients:

- 1/4 cup of organic turmeric powder

- 1 teaspoon of freshly ground black pepper

- Empty gelatin or vegetarian capsules (size 00 recommended)

- A capsule-filling machine (optional but recommended for ease)

Instructions:

1. **Mix the Ingredients:**

   o   In a small bowl, combine the turmeric powder and freshly ground black pepper. Stir thoroughly to ensure even distribution of the black pepper throughout the turmeric powder. This step is crucial because the piperine in the black pepper significantly enhances the absorption of curcumin.

2. **Fill the Capsules:**

   o   If using a capsule-filling machine, follow the manufacturer's instructions to fill the capsules with the turmeric-black pepper mixture. If you are filling the capsules by hand, carefully scoop the mixture into each capsule and seal them. Size 00 capsules are recommended as they are easy to swallow and hold an appropriate amount of the mixture.

3. **Store the Capsules:**

   o   Once all the capsules are filled, store them in an airtight container in a cool, dry place. Proper storage is essential to maintain the potency of the active ingredients.

Dosage and How to Use:

- **General Dosage:**

   o   For adults, the recommended dosage is 1 to 2 capsules (each containing approximately 500 mg of turmeric and 2.5 mg of black pepper) taken twice daily with meals. Taking the capsules with food, especially with a source of healthy fat, can further enhance the absorption of curcumin.

- **For Acute Arthritis Flare-ups:**

   o   During periods of acute pain or inflammation, the dosage can be increased to 3 capsules taken twice daily. However, it is important to monitor for any signs of gastrointestinal discomfort, as high doses of turmeric can sometimes cause stomach upset.

- **Long-term Use:**

  - These capsules can be taken consistently for long-term management of arthritis symptoms. However, it is advisable to take a break of 1-2 weeks after every 3 months of continuous use to prevent potential tolerance or reduced effectiveness.

Potential Side Effects and Precautions:

- **Gastrointestinal Issues:** Some individuals may experience mild gastrointestinal discomfort, including bloating or diarrhea, particularly at higher doses. It is advisable to start with a lower dose and gradually increase it as your body adjusts.

- **Blood Thinning:** Turmeric has natural blood-thinning properties. If you are taking blood-thinning medications or have a bleeding disorder, consult your healthcare provider before using turmeric capsules.

- **Gallbladder Issues:** Individuals with gallbladder disease or gallstones should use turmeric with caution, as it can increase bile production.

Conclusion: Homemade turmeric and black pepper capsules are a powerful natural remedy for managing arthritis. By taking advantage of turmeric's anti-inflammatory properties and black pepper's ability to enhance curcumin absorption, these capsules can significantly reduce pain and inflammation in the joints. Regular use, in combination with a healthy diet and lifestyle, can help alleviate the symptoms of arthritis and improve joint health over time.

Herbal Foot Bath for Arthritis

Arthritis often affects the joints in the feet, leading to discomfort and pain that can make walking and standing difficult. In addition to systemic treatments like turmeric capsules, localized therapies such as herbal foot baths can provide significant relief. Herbal foot baths, which combine the soothing properties of warm water with the therapeutic benefits of herbs, are an excellent way to reduce pain, inflammation, and stiffness in the feet.

Dr. Barbara O'Neill advocates for the use of natural remedies to manage arthritis symptoms, and herbal foot baths are a part of this holistic approach. The warm water in a foot bath helps to increase blood circulation to the affected area, while the herbs work to reduce inflammation, relax muscles, and alleviate pain.

Recipe: Herbal Foot Bath with Epsom Salt, Lavender, and Peppermint

Ingredients:

- 1/2 cup of Epsom salt

- 2 tablespoons of dried lavender flowers or 10 drops of lavender essential oil

- 2 tablespoons of dried peppermint leaves or 10 drops of peppermint essential oil

- 4-6 quarts of warm water (approximately 104°F to 110°F)

- A large basin or foot bath tub

Instructions:

1. **Prepare the Water:**

    o Fill a large basin or foot bath tub with warm water. The water should be comfortably warm but not scalding, ideally between 104°F to 110°F. This temperature is effective for increasing blood circulation and relieving muscle tension without causing discomfort.

2. **Add the Epsom Salt:**

    o Dissolve 1/2 cup of Epsom salt in the warm water. Epsom salt, which contains magnesium sulfate, is known for its muscle-relaxing and anti-inflammatory properties. It can help reduce swelling and ease pain in the joints.

3. **Add the Lavender and Peppermint:**

   o If using dried lavender flowers and peppermint leaves, add them directly to the water. If using essential oils, add 10 drops of each lavender and peppermint oil to the water. Lavender has calming and anti-inflammatory properties, while peppermint provides a cooling effect and helps to reduce pain.

4. **Soak Your Feet:**

   o Immerse your feet in the herbal foot bath for 20-30 minutes. During this time, relax and let the warmth and herbal properties work on your aching joints. Gently move your feet and toes to stimulate circulation and enhance the benefits of the bath.

5. **Aftercare:**

   o After soaking, dry your feet thoroughly, especially between the toes, to prevent any fungal infections. For added relief, you can apply a natural moisturizer or an anti-inflammatory balm to your feet after the bath.

Dosage and How to Use:

- **Frequency:**

  o For chronic arthritis symptoms, it is recommended to use the herbal foot bath 2-3 times a week. This frequency can help maintain reduced inflammation and pain levels in the feet and joints.

- **Duration:**

  o Each foot bath session should last between 20-30 minutes. This duration is sufficient for the herbs and Epsom salt to exert their therapeutic effects while avoiding excessive skin wrinkling or dryness.

Potential Side Effects and Precautions:

- **Skin Sensitivity:** Some individuals may have sensitive skin or allergies to essential oils. It is advisable to perform a patch test before using lavender or peppermint oils in the bath. If any irritation occurs, discontinue use or reduce the amount of essential oil.

- **Diabetes and Neuropathy:** Individuals with diabetes or neuropathy should use caution when soaking their feet. Ensure that the water is not too hot, as reduced sensation in the feet may prevent you from feeling if the water is too warm, potentially leading to burns.

Conclusion: Herbal foot baths are a simple yet effective way to manage arthritis symptoms, particularly in the feet and lower legs. By combining the therapeutic benefits of warm water, Epsom salt, lavender, and peppermint, this natural remedy can help to reduce pain, inflammation, and stiffness, allowing for greater mobility and comfort. Regular use of this remedy, along with other natural treatments, can significantly improve the quality of life for individuals suffering from arthritis

THE END

Made in the USA
Las Vegas, NV
11 September 2024

95151593R00037